SMILE WITH CONFIDENCE

The Essential Guide to Oral Hygiene

Dentist Elgiva Gabriel

Dedication

This great confidence boasting book is dedicated to everyone who will not only read this great guide, but also apply the principle in it to smile with confidence.

Table of Content

Dedication

Table of Content

Introduction

Chapter 1

Oral Hygiene: Why it Matters

Chapter 2

The Basics of Oral Hygiene: Brushing, Flossing, and More

Chapter 3

Choosing the Right Toothbrush and Toothpaste

Chapter 4

Advanced Oral Hygiene Techniques: Whitening and Straightening Your Teeth

Chapter 5

Maintaining Oral Hygiene on the Go

Chapter 6

The Role of the Dentist in Oral Health

Chapter 7

Importance of teaching good oral hygiene habits to children from an early age.

Chapter 8

Importance of maintaining good oral hygiene as you age.

Chapter 9

Common Oral Health Problems and How to Prevent Them

Chapter 10

Link between oral health and overall health.

Chapter 11

Achieving a Confident Smile: Tips and Techniques

Conclusion

A Lifetime of Healthy Teeth and Gums

Introduction

In this book, we will be exploring the importance of oral hygiene and how it affects our overall health and well-being. From brushing and flossing to visiting the dentist, we will cover all the essential steps you need to take to maintain a healthy mouth.

But taking care of your oral health isn't just about keeping your teeth and gums healthy; it's about having the confidence to smile without hesitation. When you take care of your mouth, you'll feel better about yourself and be more confident in social situations.

So, join us as we delve into the world of oral hygiene and learn how to maintain a healthy mouth and a confident smile. We'll cover everything from the basics of brushing and flossing to advanced techniques for whitening and straightening your teeth.

By the end of this book, you'll have all the knowledge and tools you need to take charge of your oral health and smile with confidence. Let's get started!

Did you know that the state of your oral health can have a significant impact on your overall health and well-being? Research has shown that there is a link between oral health and conditions such as heart disease, diabetes, and even pregnancy complications. That's why it's **so important** to take care of your mouth;

not only for the sake of your teeth and gums but for your overall health as well.

But maintaining good oral hygiene isn't always easy. It requires a consistent and thorough routine, as well as regular visits to the dentist. And let's be honest, nobody enjoys going to the dentist! But with the right knowledge and tools, taking care of your oral health can be simple and even enjoyable.

That's where this book comes in. **"Smile with Confidence: The Essential Guide to Oral Hygiene"** is here to help you understand the importance of oral hygiene and give you the tools you need to maintain a healthy mouth. Whether you're a beginner or an experienced oral health enthusiast, there's something in this book for everyone.

Throughout the pages of this book, **we'll cover topics such as:**

The basics of oral hygiene: brushing, flossing, and more

How to choose the right toothbrush and toothpaste for your needs

Tips for keeping your mouth healthy on the go

Advanced techniques for whitening and straightening your teeth

The role of the dentist in maintaining oral health

And much more!

By the end of this book, you'll have a comprehensive understanding of how to take care of your oral health and achieve a confident smile. So, let's dive in and get started!

CHAPTER 1

Oral Hygiene: Why it Matters

In this chapter, we'll be discussing the importance of oral hygiene and why it matters. First and foremost, it's important to understand that oral hygiene is about more than just keeping your teeth and gums healthy. It's about maintaining the overall health of your mouth, including your tongue, cheeks, and lips. When you take care of your oral health, you're not only preventing tooth decay and gum disease – you're also reducing your risk of developing other health problems.

Research has shown that there is a link between oral health and conditions such as heart disease, diabetes, and even pregnancy complications. Poor oral hygiene can also lead to bad breath, which can affect your social and professional relationships.

But maintaining good oral hygiene isn't always easy. It requires a consistent and thorough routine, as well as regular visits to the dentist. And let's be honest – nobody enjoys going to the dentist! But with the right knowledge and tools, taking care of your oral health can be simple and even enjoyable.

That's where this book comes in. "Smile with Confidence: The Essential Guide to Oral Hygiene" is here to help you understand the importance of oral hygiene and give you the tools you need to maintain a healthy mouth. Whether you're a beginner or an experienced oral health enthusiast, there's something in this book for everyone.

In the next few chapters, we'll be covering topics such as the basics of oral hygiene, how to choose the right toothbrush and toothpaste, and advanced techniques for whitening and straightening your teeth. We'll also be discussing the role of the dentist in maintaining oral health and how to prevent common oral health problems.

In addition to the physical health benefits of maintaining good oral hygiene, there are also mental and emotional benefits to consider. When you have healthy teeth and gums, you're more likely to feel confident in social situations. This can lead to improved relationships with others and a greater sense of overall well-being.

But if you're not taking care of your oral health, you may feel self-conscious about your smile. You may be less likely to smile or engage with others, which can lead to feelings of isolation and depression.

That's why it's so important to prioritize oral hygiene; not just for the sake of your teeth and gums, but for your overall health and well-being. With the right knowledge and tools, you can take charge of your oral health and achieve a confident, healthy smile.

In the next few chapters, we'll be exploring all the essential elements of oral hygiene, including brushing, flossing, and more. We'll also be discussing advanced techniques for whitening and straightening your teeth, as well as the role of the dentist in maintaining oral health.

So, if you're ready to learn how to take care of your oral health and achieve a confident smile, let's dive in and get started!

So, let's get started on our journey to a healthy mouth and a confident smile!

CHAPTER 2

The Basics of Oral Hygiene: Brushing, Flossing, and More

In this chapter, we'll be discussing the basics of oral hygiene – the foundation upon which a healthy mouth is built.

Let's start with brushing. Brushing your teeth at least twice a day is essential for removing plaque; a sticky film of bacteria that forms on your teeth. Plaque can lead to tooth decay and gum disease if it's not removed regularly.

To brush your teeth effectively, you'll need a toothbrush with soft bristles and toothpaste that contains fluoride. Fluoride helps to strengthen tooth enamel and prevent tooth decay.

When brushing, be sure to brush all surfaces of your teeth, including the fronts, backs, and tops. Hold your brush at a 45-degree angle to your gums and use gentle circular motions. Aim to brush for at least two minutes – you can use a timer or a two-minute song to help you keep track.

Flossing is another essential aspect of oral hygiene. Flossing helps to remove plaque and food particles that your toothbrush can't reach. It's important to floss at least once a day, ideally before you brush your teeth.

To floss effectively, use about 18 inches of floss and wind it around your middle fingers. Hold the floss tightly between your thumb and forefinger and use a gentle back-and-forth motion to slide it between your teeth. Don't forget to floss behind your back teeth!

In addition to brushing and flossing, it's also important to use mouthwash and replace your toothbrush every three to four months. These simple steps can help to keep your mouth healthy and prevent oral health problems.

That's it for the basics of oral hygiene! In the next few chapters, we'll be discussing advanced techniques for maintaining a healthy mouth, as well as the role of the dentist in oral health.

Remember, taking care of your oral hygiene is essential for maintaining a healthy mouth and a confident smile. By following these basic steps, you'll be well on your way to achieving both.

In addition to brushing and flossing, there are a few other steps you can take to maintain good oral hygiene. **Here are a few more tips:**

Use mouthwash: Mouthwash can help to kill bacteria and freshen your breath. Look for a mouthwash that contains fluoride to help strengthen tooth enamel and prevent tooth decay.

Replace your toothbrush regularly: It's important to replace your toothbrush every three to four months, or sooner if the bristles become frayed. A worn-out toothbrush won't be as effective at removing plaque and can even irritate your gums.

Avoid sugary foods and drinks: Sugary foods and drinks can contribute to tooth decay. Try to limit your intake of these types of foods and drinks, especially between meals.

Drink plenty of water: Water helps to rinse away food particles and bacteria from your mouth. Aim for at least eight glasses of water per day to help keep your mouth clean and healthy.

Avoid tobacco products: Tobacco products, including cigarettes and chewing tobacco, can contribute to oral health problems such as gum disease and tooth loss. If you use tobacco products, consider quitting to improve your oral health.

By following these simple steps in addition to brushing and flossing, you can maintain a healthy mouth and a confident smile. Remember, good oral hygiene is essential for overall health and well-being – so make it a priority!

CHAPTER 3

Choosing the Right Toothbrush and Toothpaste

Welcome to chapter 3 of "Smile with Confidence: The Essential Guide to Oral Hygiene"! In this chapter, we'll be discussing how to choose the right toothbrush and toothpaste for your needs.

When it comes to toothbrushes, there are a few key factors to consider:

1. **Bristles:** Look for a toothbrush with soft or medium bristles. Hard bristles can be too abrasive and

damage your tooth enamel and gums.

2. **Size and shape:** Choose a toothbrush that fits comfortably in your hand and can reach all areas of your mouth. A smaller toothbrush may be easier to maneuver in tight spaces, such as between your back teeth.

3. **Type:** There are several types of toothbrushes to choose from, including manual, electric, and sonic. Each type has its pros and cons, so consider your needs and preferences when making a decision.

When it comes to toothpaste, there are also a few key factors to consider:

1. **Fluoride:** Fluoride helps to strengthen tooth enamel and prevent tooth decay. Look for toothpaste that contains fluoride.

2. **Sensitivity:** If you have sensitive teeth, look for a toothpaste that is specifically formulated for sensitivity. These kinds of toothpaste typically contain ingredients that help to block the sensation of sensitivity.

3. **Flavor:** Toothpaste comes in a variety of flavors, so choose one that you enjoy. Some people prefer minty flavors, while others prefer fruity flavors.

4. **Special needs:** If you have specific oral health needs, such as gum disease or staining, there are available that are formulated specifically for these needs.

By choosing the right toothbrush and toothpaste, you'll be better equipped to maintain a healthy mouth and a confident smile. In the next few chapters, we'll be discussing advanced techniques for maintaining a healthy mouth, as well as the role of the dentist in oral health.

Remember, good oral hygiene is essential for overall health and well-being – so make it a priority!

In addition to the factors mentioned above, there are a few other things to

1. **Brand:** There are many different brands of toothbrushes and toothpaste to choose from. Consider reading reviews and looking for recommendations from trusted sources to help you make a decision.

2. **Price:** Toothbrushes and toothpaste come in a range of prices. Decide on a budget and look for a product that fits within it. Remember, the most expensive option isn't always the best – sometimes a more affordable option can work just as well.

3. **Eco-friendliness:** If you're interested in using eco-friendly products, there are toothbrushes and toothpaste available that are

made with environmentally-friendly materials.

By considering these additional factors, you can choose a toothbrush and toothpaste that are right for you and your needs. Remember to replace your toothbrush every three to four months and choose a toothpaste that contains fluoride to help maintain a healthy mouth and a confident smile.

CHAPTER 4

Advanced Oral Hygiene Techniques: Whitening and Straightening Your Teeth

Welcome to chapter 4 of "Smile with Confidence: The Essential Guide to Oral Hygiene"! In this chapter, we'll be discussing advanced oral hygiene techniques for whitening and straightening your teeth.

Let's start with teeth whitening. Many people want to have a brighter, more radiant smile, and teeth whitening is a popular way to achieve this. There are several options for teeth whitening, including:

1. **Over-the-counter products:** There are many over-the-counter teeth whitening products available, including strips, gels, and trays. These products can be effective, but results may vary.

2. **Professional teeth whitening:** Professional teeth whitening is performed by a dental professional and typically involves the use of a stronger bleaching agent. This option tends to be more expensive than over-the-counter products, but it may produce better results.

3. **Natural teeth whitening:** If you're looking for a more natural option, there are a few things you can try at home. Brushing your teeth with baking soda and hydrogen peroxide can help to remove surface stains.

In addition to teeth whitening, another advanced oral hygiene technique is teeth straightening. There are several options for straightening teeth, including:

- **Braces:** Braces are a traditional method of straightening teeth and are typically recommended for more severe misalignment. Braces use metal brackets and wires to slowly move the teeth into their correct positions.

- **Clear aligners:** Clear aligners, such as Invisalign, are a newer method of straightening teeth. These aligners are made of a clear plastic material and are virtually invisible when worn. Clear aligners are typically more expensive than braces, but they are more discreet and may be more comfortable for some people.

- **Retainers:** Retainers are a type of appliance that is worn after teeth have been straightened to help keep them in their correct positions. Retainers can be removable or fixed, and they are typically worn at night.

By choosing the right teeth whitening or straightening option for your needs, you can achieve a brighter, more confident smile. Remember, good oral hygiene is essential for overall health and well-being – so make it a priority!

Some Tips to Consider

Consider your budget: Teeth whitening and straightening can be expensive, so it's important to consider your budget when deciding on a treatment option. While professional teeth whitening and clear aligners tend to be more expensive, they may produce better results.

Talk to your dentist: Before starting any teeth whitening or straightening treatment, it's a good idea to talk to your dentist. Your dentist can assess your oral health and recommend the best option for your needs.

Follow instructions: If you're using an over-the-counter teeth whitening product or wearing aligners or braces, be sure to follow the instructions carefully. This will help to ensure the best possible results.

Practice good oral hygiene: While teeth whitening and straightening treatments can improve the appearance of your teeth, it's important to remember that good oral hygiene is essential for maintaining healthy teeth and gums. Be sure to brush, floss, and use mouthwash regularly to keep your mouth healthy.

By following these tips, you can achieve a brighter, straighter smile and maintain good oral hygiene. With the right knowledge and tools, you can take charge of your oral health and achieve a confident smile that lasts a lifetime.

CHAPTER 5

Maintaining Oral Hygiene on the Go

Welcome to chapter 5 of "Smile with Confidence: The Essential Guide to Oral Hygiene"! In this chapter, we'll be discussing how to maintain oral hygiene when you're on the go.

Maintaining good oral hygiene can be a challenge when you're away from home, but it's important to make an effort to keep your mouth clean and healthy no matter where you are.

Here are a few tips for maintaining oral hygiene on the go:

1. **Pack a travel-sized toothbrush and toothpaste:** Keep a small toothbrush and toothpaste with you when you're traveling so you can brush your teeth after meals. You may also want to pack a travel-sized mouthwash for an extra fresh feeling.

2. **Carry floss with you:** Floss is small and easy to pack, so be sure to carry some with you when you're on the go. You can floss in the car, on a plane, or in a public bathroom – anywhere you have access to water.

3. **Drink water:** Water helps to rinse away food particles and bacteria from your mouth. Keep a water

bottle with you when you're on the go to help keep your mouth clean and hydrated.

4. Avoid sugary foods and drinks.

In addition to the tips mentioned above, here are a few more ways to maintain oral hygiene when you're on the go:

- **Choose healthy snacks:** When you're away from home, it can be tempting to grab convenience foods that are high in sugar. However, these types of foods can contribute to tooth decay. Instead, opt for healthy snacks such as fruits, vegetables, and nuts.

- **Use a tongue scraper:** A tongue scraper can help to remove bacteria and food particles from your tongue, which can help to freshen your breath. You can find tongue scrapers at most drugstores or online.

- **Use disposable toothbrushes:** If you're traveling and don't have access to a sink to rinse your toothbrush, consider using disposable toothbrushes. These toothbrushes come pre-pasted and can be thrown away after use.

By following these tips, you can maintain good oral hygiene even when you're on the go. Remember, good oral hygiene is essential for overall health and well-being. So, make it a priority no matter where you are!

CHAPTER 6

The Role of the Dentist in Oral Health

Welcome to chapter 6 of "Smile with Confidence: The Essential Guide to Oral Hygiene"! In this chapter, we'll be discussing the role of the dentist in maintaining oral health.

While brushing, flossing, and using mouthwash are essential for maintaining good oral hygiene, **regular visits to the dentist are also important.** Your dentist can help to identify and treat any oral health problems in their early stages, which can help to prevent more serious issues from developing.

During a dental checkup, your dentist will examine your teeth, gums, and mouth for any problems. They may take x-rays to get a better look at your teeth and identify any issues that may not be visible on the surface.

Your dentist may also clean your teeth to remove plaque and tartar; hard deposits of bacteria that can lead to gum disease and tooth decay. This process, called scaling and polishing, can help to keep your teeth and gums healthy.

In addition to checkups and cleanings, your dentist may also recommend other treatments to maintain your oral health.

These treatments may include fillings, crowns, or root canals.

It's recommended that you visit the dentist at least twice a year for a checkup and cleaning. However, if you have any specific oral health concerns, you may need to visit more frequently.

By visiting the dentist regularly and following their recommendations, you can maintain good oral hygiene and achieve a healthy, confident smile. Remember, good oral hygiene is essential for overall health and well-being. So, make it a priority!

In addition to regular checkups and cleanings, there are a few other ways that your dentist can help you maintain good oral hygiene:

1. **Oral cancer screening:** Oral cancer can be serious and can be difficult to detect in its early stages. During a dental checkup, your dentist will examine your mouth, tongue, and throat for any signs of oral cancer. If they suspect a problem, they may recommend further testing.

2. **Gum disease treatment:** Gum disease, or periodontitis, is an infection of the gums that can lead to tooth loss if left untreated. Your dentist can diagnose and treat gum disease to help prevent further damage to your teeth and gums.

3. **Orthodontic treatment:** If you have misaligned teeth or an improper bite, your dentist may recommend orthodontic treatment to correct these issues. Orthodontic treatment can include braces, clear aligners, or other appliances that help to straighten your teeth.

By working with your dentist and following their recommendations, you can maintain good oral hygiene and achieve a healthy, confident smile. Remember, good oral hygiene is essential for overall health and well-being. So, make it a priority!

CHAPTER 7

Importance of teaching good oral hygiene habits to children from an early age.

Welcome to chapter 7 of "Smile with Confidence: The Essential Guide to Oral Hygiene"! In this chapter, we'll be discussing the importance of teaching good oral hygiene habits to children from an early age.

Good oral hygiene is essential for overall health and well-being, and it's important to start teaching good habits to children from an early age.

Here are a few tips for teaching good oral hygiene habits to children:

1. **Start early:** Children should start brushing and flossing as soon as they have teeth. You can help your child brush their teeth by using a soft-bristled toothbrush and a small amount of toothpaste.

2. **Make it fun:** Children may be more likely to brush their teeth if it's an enjoyable activity. Consider using a timer to make brushing a game, or let your child choose their toothbrush and toothpaste.

3. **Set a good example:** Children often model their behavior after their parents, so it's important to set a good example by brushing and flossing regularly yourself.

4. **Visit the dentist regularly:** Regular visits to the dentist can help to establish good oral hygiene habits and identify any potential problems early on.

By teaching good oral hygiene habits to your children from an early age, you can help them maintain good oral health and a confident smile for a lifetime. Remember, good oral hygiene is essential for overall health and well-being. So, make it a priority!

In addition to the tips mentioned above, here are a few more ways to help your children maintain good oral hygiene:

- **Encourage healthy eating habits:** Sugary foods and drinks can contribute to tooth decay, so it's important to encourage your children to eat a healthy, balanced diet. Offer them plenty of fruits, vegetables, and water to help keep their teeth and gums healthy.

- **Use fluoride toothpaste:** Fluoride helps to strengthen tooth enamel and prevent tooth decay. Use toothpaste that contains fluoride to help protect your child's teeth.

- **Supervise brushing:** Children under the age of 8 should be supervised while brushing to ensure that they are brushing properly and not swallowing too much toothpaste.

- **Talk to your dentist:** If you have any concerns about your child's oral hygiene or development, be sure to talk to your dentist. They can provide guidance and recommendations to help your child maintain good oral health.

By following these tips, you can help your children develop good oral hygiene habits that will last a lifetime. Remember, good oral hygiene is essential for overall health and well-being. So, make it a priority!

CHAPTER 8

Importance of maintaining good oral hygiene as you age.

Welcome to chapter 8 of "Smile with Confidence: The Essential Guide to Oral Hygiene"! In this chapter, we'll be discussing the importance of maintaining good oral hygiene as you age.

As we get older, our oral health needs can change. It's important to continue practicing good oral hygiene habits and visiting the dentist regularly to maintain a healthy mouth as you age.

Here are a few tips for maintaining good oral hygiene as you age:

Brush and floss regularly: It's important to brush your teeth twice a day and floss daily to remove plaque and food particles from your mouth. This can help to prevent tooth decay and gum disease.

Use fluoride toothpaste: Fluoride helps to strengthen tooth enamel and prevent tooth decay. Use toothpaste that contains fluoride to help protect your teeth.

Use a soft-bristled toothbrush: As we age, our gums may become more sensitive. A soft-bristled toothbrush can be gentler on the gums and help to prevent irritation.

Consider using an electric toothbrush: An electric toothbrush can be more effective at removing plaque and may be easier for some people to use as they age.

By following these tips, you can maintain good oral hygiene and a healthy mouth as you age. Remember, good oral hygiene is essential for overall health and well-being.

In addition to the tips mentioned above, here are a few more ways to maintain good oral hygiene as you age:

Stay hydrated: Dry mouth is a common issue for older adults, which can lead to tooth decay and gum disease. It's important to drink plenty of water to help keep your mouth hydrated.

Use mouthwash: Mouthwash can help to kill bacteria and freshen your breath. Consider using a mouthwash that contains fluoride to help protect your teeth.

Don't neglect your dentures: If you wear dentures, be sure to clean them regularly to remove food particles and bacteria. Soak them in a denture cleaner or use a soft-bristled toothbrush and toothpaste to clean them.

Visit the dentist regularly: Regular visits to the dentist can help to identify any potential issues early on and keep your mouth healthy.

By following these tips, you can maintain good oral hygiene and a healthy mouth as you age. Remember, good oral hygiene is essential for overall health and well-being. So, make it a priority!

CHAPTER 9

Common Oral Health Problems and How to Prevent Them

Good oral health is essential for overall health and well-being. It is important to be aware of the most common oral health problems and take steps to prevent them. Oral health is an essential part of overall health and well-being.

Some of the most common oral health problems include:

- ★ **Tooth Decay:** Tooth decay is a common problem caused by bacteria in the mouth that produce acid that breaks down the enamel and dentin of a tooth. This can lead to cavities, which can cause pain and infection if left untreated.

- **Prevention:** To prevent tooth decay, it is important to practice good oral hygiene by brushing your teeth twice a day with fluoride toothpaste, flossing daily, and using mouthwash to kill bacteria. Limiting sugary and acidic foods and drinks, as well as visiting your dentist regularly for check-ups and cleanings, can also help prevent tooth decay.

★ **Gum Disease:** Gum disease is an infection of the gums that can cause inflammation, swelling, and bleeding. If left untreated, it can lead to tooth loss and other serious health problems.

• **Prevention:** To prevent gum disease, it is important to practice good oral hygiene, including brushing, flossing, and using mouthwash regularly. Visiting your dentist for regular check-ups and cleanings is also important. Additionally, avoiding smoking and limiting alcohol consumption can help prevent gum disease.

★ **Bad Breath:** Bad breath is caused by bacteria in the mouth that produce unpleasant odors. Certain foods and drinks, such as garlic and coffee, can also contribute to bad breath.

- **Prevention:** To prevent bad breath, it is important to practice good oral hygiene, including brushing, flossing, and using mouthwash regularly. Chewing sugar-free gum and avoiding sugary and acidic foods and drinks can also help prevent bad breath. Drinking plenty of water and avoiding alcohol and tobacco can also help.

- ★ **Tooth Sensitivity:** Tooth sensitivity is a common problem that causes discomfort or pain when eating or drinking hot, cold, or sweet foods and drinks.

- **Prevention:** To prevent tooth sensitivity, it is important to practice good oral hygiene and avoid brushing too hard, as well as avoid excessive consumption of sugary and acidic foods and drinks. Using toothpaste specifically designed for sensitive teeth can also help. If you have persistent tooth sensitivity, it is best to see your dentist for a diagnosis and treatment plan.

★ **Tooth Wear:** Tooth wear is a common problem that occurs due to friction, grinding, or erosion of the tooth's surface. This can cause pain, sensitivity, and aesthetic concerns.

• **Prevention:** To prevent tooth wear, it is important to avoid excessive grinding and clenching of the teeth, and to protect the teeth from erosion caused by acidic foods and drinks. Wearing a night guard if you grind your teeth at night can also help. If you have symptoms of tooth wear, it is best to see your dentist for a diagnosis and treatment plan.

★ **Oral Cancer:** Oral cancer is a serious condition that affects the mouth, tongue, or throat. It can cause pain, swelling, and changes in the way that you speak, eat or breathe.

• **Prevention:** To prevent oral cancer, it is important to avoid tobacco and excessive alcohol consumption, as these are known risk factors. Regular dental check-ups can also help to detect oral cancer in its early stages when it is most treatable.

★ **Mouth Sores:** Mouth sores, also known as canker sores, are small, painful ulcers that can occur in the mouth. They can be caused by a variety of factors, including injury, infection, or autoimmune disorders.

• **Prevention:** To prevent mouth sores, it is important to maintain good oral hygiene, avoid acidic and spicy foods, and limit stress. If you have persistent or severe mouth sores, it is best to see your dentist for a diagnosis and treatment plan.

In addition to these common oral health problems, **other issues such as jaw pain, temporomandibular joint disorder (TMJ), and sleep apnea** can also affect oral health. To maintain a healthy mouth and body, it is important to practice good oral hygiene, see your dentist regularly, and make healthy lifestyle choices. Good oral hygiene, regular dental check-ups, and healthy lifestyle choices can help prevent common oral health problems and ensure a lifetime of healthy teeth and gums.

CHAPTER 10

Link between oral health and overall health.

Welcome to chapter 10 of "Smile with Confidence: The Essential Guide to Oral Hygiene"! In this chapter, we'll be discussing the link between oral health and overall health.

Good oral hygiene is essential for overall health and well-being. Studies have shown that there is a link between oral health and other health issues, such as heart disease, diabetes, and pregnancy complications.

Here are a few ways that good oral hygiene can affect the rest of your body:

1. **Oral bacteria can enter the bloodstream:** Bacteria in your mouth can enter your bloodstream through your gums, leading to inflammation in other parts of your body. This inflammation has been linked to heart disease, diabetes, and other health issues.

2. **Poor oral hygiene can affect pregnancy outcomes:** Studies have shown that pregnant women with gum disease are more likely to have premature, low birth weight babies.

3. **Good oral hygiene can improve overall health:** By maintaining good oral hygiene, you can help to reduce the risk of oral health problems and the associated health issues.

By following good oral hygiene habits and visiting the dentist regularly, you can help to maintain good oral health and overall health and well-being. Remember, good oral hygiene is essential for overall health and well-being.

In addition to the points mentioned above, here are a few more ways that good oral hygiene can affect the rest of your body:

Good oral hygiene can improve self-esteem: People with good oral hygiene tend to have a more confident smile, which can improve self-esteem and social interactions.

Poor oral hygiene can affect mental health: Studies have shown that people with poor oral hygiene are more likely to experience anxiety and depression.

Good oral hygiene can improve respiratory health: Bacteria from the mouth can be inhaled into the lungs, leading to respiratory infections. Good oral hygiene can help to reduce the risk of respiratory infections.

Poor oral hygiene can affect sleep quality: People with poor oral hygiene may be more likely to experience sleep apnea, a condition in which breathing is disrupted during sleep.

By following good oral hygiene habits and visiting the dentist regularly, you can help to maintain good oral health and overall health and well-being. Remember, good oral hygiene is essential for overall health and well-being. So, make it a priority!

CHAPTER 11

Achieving a Confident Smile: Tips and Techniques

A confident smile can have a significant impact on one's self-esteem and overall well-being.

Here are some tips and techniques to help you achieve a confident smile:

Practice Good Oral Hygiene: Good oral hygiene is essential for maintaining healthy teeth and gums, which is the foundation for a confident smile. Brush your teeth twice a day with fluoride toothpaste, floss daily, and use mouthwash to kill bacteria. Regular dental check-ups and cleanings are also important to ensure that your oral health is in good condition.

Brighten Your Smile: If your teeth are discolored or stained, you may feel self-conscious about your smile. Teeth whitening treatments, such as at-home kits or in-office procedures, can help brighten your smile and boost your confidence.

Straighten Your Teeth: If you have crooked or misaligned teeth, orthodontic treatment, such as braces or Invisalign, can help straighten your teeth and improve your smile.

Repair Dental Issues: If you have dental issues, such as cavities, broken teeth, or missing teeth, it can affect your confidence and your smile. Repairing these issues with dental treatments, such as fillings, crowns, bridges, or implants, can help improve your smile and boost your confidence.

Improve Your Lip Health: If your lips are dry, chapped, or wrinkled, it can affect the appearance of your smile. Keeping your lips moisturized and protected from the sun can help improve their appearance and enhance your smile.

Practice Confident Body Language: Confident body language, such as standing tall, making eye contact, and smiling, can help you feel more confident about your smile. Practicing confident body language can also make you appear more approachable and friendly to others.

Maintain a Healthy Diet: Your diet plays a crucial role in the health of your teeth and gums. Consuming a balanced diet that is rich in vitamins, minerals, and nutrients can help support the health of your oral tissues. Additionally, avoiding sugary and acidic foods and drinks can help prevent tooth decay and gum disease.

Consider Dental Procedures: In addition to orthodontic treatments, several cosmetic dental procedures can help improve the appearance of your smile. For example, veneers can be used to correct issues such as chipped, stained, or misaligned teeth. Bonding can be used to repair small chips or cracks in the teeth. And dental implants can be used to replace missing teeth and restore the function of your bite.

Seek Professional Treatment: If you have concerns about your smile, it is important to seek professional treatment. A dentist or orthodontist can evaluate your oral health and develop a personalized treatment plan to help you achieve your smile goals. They can also provide you with the guidance and support you need to make informed decisions about your dental care.

Practice Positive Self-Talk: Finally, practicing positive self-talk can help you build confidence in your smile. Focusing on the positive aspects of your smile, such as your healthy teeth and gums, can help you feel more confident about your smile. If you struggle with negative self-talk, consider working with a therapist or counselor to help you develop a more positive mindset.

Note that there are many tips and techniques to help you achieve a confident smile. From practicing good oral hygiene to repairing dental issues, there are many steps you can take to improve your smile and boost your confidence. Additionally, it is important to work with a dentist or orthodontist to develop a personalized plan to achieve your smile goals.

Don't forget, achieving a confident smile requires a combination of good oral hygiene, healthy lifestyle choices, and professional dental treatment. By following these tips and techniques, you can achieve a healthy and confident smile that will last a lifetime. Additionally, working with a dentist or orthodontist can help you develop a personalized plan to achieve your smile goals and ensure that you receive the best possible dental care.

CONCLUSION

A Lifetime of Healthy Teeth and Gums

In this guide, we have explored the importance of oral hygiene and the steps you can take to achieve and maintain a healthy smile. From practicing good oral hygiene to seeking professional treatment, there are many ways to ensure that your teeth and gums remain healthy and functional throughout your lifetime.

Achieving and maintaining good oral health requires a lifelong commitment to taking care of your teeth and gums. It is important to establish a routine for brushing and flossing, to visit your dentist regularly for check-ups and cleanings, and to make healthy lifestyle choices that support the health of your oral tissues.

It is also important to seek professional treatment if you have any concerns about your smile or oral health. A dentist or orthodontist can provide you with the guidance and support you need to make informed decisions about your dental care and to achieve your smile goals.

In conclusion, a lifetime of healthy teeth and gums is achievable with the right combination of good oral hygiene, healthy lifestyle choices, and professional dental care. By following the tips and techniques outlined in this guide, you can smile with confidence and enjoy the many benefits of a healthy and functional bite. So, go ahead and start your journey to a confident smile today!